LOW BLOOD PRESSURE

LOW BLOOD PRESSURE

TRISTAN EVERGREEN

CONTENTS

Introduction

Blood pressure is defined as the pressure of blood on the walls of arteries or when the heart contracts and relaxes. Blood pressure is measured in millimeters of mercury. Systolic pressure is the numerator and diastolic pressure is the denominator. The normal range of blood pressure for an adult should be 120/80. When it is lower than 90/60, it is likely that the individual is suffering from hypotension or low blood pressure. A low blood pressure causes the body to be deprived of oxygen because it becomes difficult for the blood to reach various parts of the body, especially the brain and heart. And when this happens, the individual is said to be weak, dizzy, and may faint.

In assessing hypotension, three components are considered: blood pressure decreases, failing heart, hypovolemia, slow heartbeat (bradycardia), or low systemic vascular resistance. Orthostatic hypotension occurs in the body when a person moves from a lying to a sitting or standing position. At this time, one may feel dizzy and subsequently faint. This is regarded as orthostatic hypotension. The diagnosis of hypotension is done after taking the personal and family history of the individual because some from certain families are even born with hypotension. A physical examination is carried out as well, together with some advanced testing like blood tests. There are cases where the individuals are not experiencing problems and therefore do not need treatment. If there are cases, treatment may include distinguishing and treating the underlying condition. There are several factors, among which are symptoms and causes associated with hypotension, that need to be addressed.

Chapter 1: Understanding Low Blood Pressure

In recent years, the frequency of low blood pressure-related diseases has significantly increased, which urges closer attention to and improved understanding of low blood pressure. This chapter introduces low blood pressure, including its definition and classification, the normal ranges of blood pressure, and common methods for blood pressure measurement, which provide a basis for the following chapters leading to a comprehensive understanding of low blood pressure.

Low blood pressure is a common but frequently overlooked issue in clinical settings. On the pathway to the final stage of hypotension severe enough to require treatment, physiologic changes in the body are complicated. Due to inadequate blood flow to tissues, various organs and structures can be directly impacted by hypotension, rendering the patient symptomatic in multiple aspects. Furthermore, the substantial decline in central perfusion pressure increases the risk of an individual's cardiovascular function becoming dangerous.

Definition and Classification

It is generally agreed that reference to a medical condition as being "hypotension" entails that the arterial pressure is exceedingly low. There is, however, no agreement of opinion as to the numerical definition of hypotension. In the seminal study, various criteria were used to define low blood pressure (BP; considered to be <90 or <80mmHg), and this is also reflected in the literature. Hypotension can be classified into primarily four categories like - orthostatic hypotensive symptoms, orthostatic hypotension without hypotensive symptoms, neurally mediated hypotension, and anti-hypertensive drug-induced hypotension.

Various authors have proposed different terminologies to describe different aspects of hypotension. However, in such a scenario, there develops a conceptual confusion, and these conditions are treated separately when they are clubbed together in actual. In the context of India, hypotension is a common and trivial symptom that is associated with strenuous physical activity, especially in farmers and laborers, who are more prone to dehydration. Other common settings in which hypotension is observed include persons fasting for long durations, malnourished persons, people suffering from infectious diseases and children with acute illnesses. Hatha Yoga, an indigenous mode of physical exercise, is also known to reduce BP and the autonomic arousability. Since the meaning of hypotension has not been clearly conceptualized, these clinical conditions have been treated separately by different scientific communities.

Normal Blood Pressure Ranges

Normal blood pressure is defined as a systolic blood pressure of less than 120 mm Hg and a diastolic blood pressure of less than 80 mm Hg. Blood pressure fluctuates within each day. It is usually lower while someone is sleeping or doing activities like reading or watching television. While someone is exercising or under stress, it rises. It can also rise when someone is in pain. Blood pressure normally increases from early childhood to adult years. Depending on age, gender, and health conditions, appropriate ranges may vary. High blood pressure, or hypertension, refers to systolic blood pressure higher than 130 mm Hg and a diastolic blood pressure higher than 89 mm Hg. The risk of heart disease or stroke increases when blood pressure is high. The risks of the potential harmful effects of high blood pressure may be higher with additional risk factors.

Correspondingly, if either number is below the threshold and, in particular, if the lower number is below the normal range of 80, it would be defined as having low blood pressure. Low blood pressure means either of the systolic blood pressure numbers drops to 90 mmHg or less, or the diastolic blood pressure numbers drop to 60 mmHg or less. If the systolic number is coupled with a lower diastolic number, it tends to cause kidney failure because the kidney was not able to supply the body with the quality of blood it needs.

How Blood Pressure is Measured

How blood pressure is measured Standard methods for blood pressure measurement in clinical settings help diagnose high blood pressure (hypertension), evaluate its effect on your circulation, as well as monitor the effects of treatment. Blood pressure is measured using millimeters of mercury (mm Hg) to describe the amount of pressure in the systolic and diastolic chambers of the heart. This is typically written as a ratio in the form of 120/80 mm Hg. When your heart beats, it contracts and pushes blood through the arteries to the rest of your body, and your blood pressure goes into the systolic phase. It is the highest blood pressure in your arteries. When your heart rests between beats, your blood pressure drops into the diastolic phase. It is the low blood pressure in your arteries.

Blood pressure measurements are not a complete description of a person's health. Diastolic blood pressure less than 60 mm Hg is generally not an immediate concern for most people unless they have symptoms such as dizziness, fainting, or chest pain. Orthostatic hypotension refers to a sudden blood pressure drop when a person stands up from a sitting position. Dehydration, some medications, and neurologic disorders can cause orthostatic hypotension. Symptoms of low blood pressure and low blood volume may also occur after standing up quickly or in severely dehydrated, ill, hospitalized people. Blood pressure is typically measured to determine the horizontal artery pressure on the right and left sides. It is important to measure blood pressure in both arms to ensure blood pressure equality because the vertical arteries of some people have significantly different pressures.

Chapter 2: Causes of Low Blood Pressure

Abnormalities in the blood or health issues can cause blood pressure that is too low and is a common condition. A lack of contractions functioning correctly or enough volume can cause low blood pressure. The causes of low blood pressure can be from lower volume of blood and dehydration in healthy people without any other medical condition. Blood volume is low when there is concurrence of enhanced losses, increased movement, or inadequate ingestion, or it may be from vasodilation or overexpansion of blood vessels. When arteries and veins widen to a greater extent than normal, blood pressure can get too low, which can lead to hypotension. Low pressure of the blood can result as well as danger to hypertensive people. Another cause of low blood pressure is the septicaemia known as reduced pressure of the blood.

There are also many medicines that can cause low blood pressure. The kidney a person has can also be the source of low blood pressure in which a lot of salt may be chopped off. Hormonal causes are also likely explanation. When the medical flow through arteries is decreased, the blood pressure of the person will fade. The same is true when the amount of blood in veins or the person's entire quantity is decreased or the arteries anterior carrier dilated too much. When the blood seems unable to prevent and contact the bloodstream from settling down, it is often called venous pool formation. Any combination of the above would lead to drops in BP. When the flow of blood to the heart is decreased, heart muscle starts to hurt.

Dehydration and Blood Loss

As previously highlighted, the volume of blood in the body needs to be maintained to meet the heart's capacity to distribute oxygen and nutrients. Nonetheless, issues such as dehydration and blood loss can severely reduce the heart's ability to pump sufficient blood. Dehydration involves the loss of a significant amount of plasma, the liquid portion of the blood, from the intravascular space. This accounts for 5% of a person's weight loss. In adults, such a loss results in an increase in heart rate by at least 15–20% starting from 120 beats per minute or an absolute heart rate of more than 100 beats per minute. Dehydration can be caused by different factors, such as infections, medications, excessive sweating, and other issues that reduce fluid intake.

On the other hand, blood loss (hypovolemia) involves the loss of cells or plasma from the blood. Such could occur due to injuries and, occasionally, ulcerations in the stomach or the use of non-steroidal anti-inflammatory drugs (NSAIDs). When the volume of blood is reduced by 10% from the baseline level, the heart rate increases, stroke volume decreases, total peripheral resistance increases, and blood pressure falls. Blood pressure drops in proportion to the amount of blood lost, which could be dangerous for the body. Maintaining blood volume is essential in managing low blood pressure, such as avoiding factors that could reduce its volume is important in preventing episodes of low blood pressure.

Heart Conditions

• Heart attack: Blockage in the coronary artery leading to reduced oxygen levels may damage the heart. In such a situation, the damaged heart will be unable to supply enough blood, causing low blood pressure. • Slow heart rate: Slow heart rate (bradycardia) due to electrical conduction problems, heart block, or sick sinus syndrome may lead to a reduced cardiac output, thus resulting in low blood pressure. • Heart valve problems: Causes backflow of blood (regurgitation) or leads to valve not opening properly, thus leading to low blood pressure. • Amyloidosis: Amyloidosis causes the accumulation of abnormal proteins in the heart and other organs. Myeloma proteins build up in tissues and organs, leading to heart failure which eventually causes low blood pressure. • Pericarditis: Fluid accumulation and inflammation in the sac around the heart (pericardium) may lead to low blood pressure due to the absence of necessary ventricular contraction.

Low blood pressure occurs as a result of conditions that decrease total blood volume or the ability of blood vessels to constrict effectively, which decreases cardiac output enough to reduce blood pressure. Low blood pressure is common in patients with heart failure. Blood pressure can be lowest when heart muscle is weak because the heart is unable to pump enough blood to meet the body's needs. This situation can be compounded by the use of medications such as beta-blockers that are used to treat heart failure, which can reduce blood pressure too much. There are many causes of low blood pressure unique to the heart including arrhythmias, pericarditis, amyloidosis, acute heart attack, and heart valve disease.

Endocrine Disorders

In the endocrine system disorders, the patient is prone to various diseases related to adrenal and thyroid diseases. Hormones secreted by these organs have a direct effect on the cardiovascular system and the degree of these disorders. Adrenal gland disorders cause excessive adrenal hormone secretion. If high blood pressure is high, and if low blood pressure is low. In the case of a thyroid disorder, an anomaly (abnormal) will be low in both systolic and diastolic blood pressures. An increase in thyroid hormones directly increases cardiac injury, cardiac output, and blood pressure. Furthermore, these hormones increase energy consumption due to an increase in body metabolism. In this table, the person will have palpitation complaints, the rapid rate of movement, weight loss, and will seek a doctor with complaints. In the treatments of such cases, first of all, endocrine disorders are corrected.

In cases of low blood pressure, cardiovascular causes and additionally, hormonal causes should be considered together. In the regulation of cardiovascular events with the help of hormonal mechanisms (especially adrenal, which has a direct relationship with the heart) against endocrine disorders, low blood pressure can be tried. Since these hormones are secreted from endocrine glands called adrenal and thyroid glands, even if low blood pressure occurs, endocrine glands should first be checked together with the cardiovascular system.

Chapter 3: Symptoms and Complications

Symptoms The most common symptom of hypotension is dizziness or lightheadedness, especially when shifting from lying to sitting or standing. Other symptoms may include:

- Blurred vision - Fainting or syncope (temporary loss of consciousness) - Fast, shallow breathing - Fatigue - Nausea - Difficulty focusing, depression, or irritability

Unusual symptoms or excessive drop in blood pressure can be life-threatening. These may include:

- Chest pain - Heart palpitations - Shortness of breath - Numbness or tingling in the extremities - Loss of appetite - Unexplained weight loss or loss of body mass

Complications Decreases in blood pressure can cause sudden falls, which result in acute, and often serious, physical impacts. As such, people with this condition are more susceptible to:

- Falls and fractures - Stroke - Heart attack - Problems during pregnancy

In more severe cases, such as sepsis or trauma, severe drops in pressure can result in life-threatening outcomes, including:

- Heart or multiorgan failure - Kidney damage or failure - Pulmonary embolism (blood clot to the lungs) - Brain injury (due to hypoxemia or lack of oxygen to the brain)

Common Symptoms

One of the issues with low blood pressure is that many people may experience no symptoms at all unless their blood pressure drops 20% or more below their normal level. In many cases, those symptoms may be tied to an underlying condition that is causing the fall in blood pressure. Some of the symptoms that may occur alongside the low blood pressure because of this include the following:

* Dizziness or fainting. * Thirst or dehydration. * Nausea. * Lack of concentration. * Blurred vision. * Rapid, shallow breathing. * Fatigue and general lack of energy. * Confusion, particularly in relation to time and place.

It is important to note, however, that there are also many medications that can cause low blood pressure as a side effect. In some cases, individuals may still feel as though their blood pressure is raised, because they feel more tired due to fatigue from an underlying condition or medication and conflate the two sensations. In some rarer cases, patients may sustain more severe conditions, like heart palpitations, or even seizures. In these cases, a person should seek emergency medical attention to have the condition diagnosed and treated.

Potential Complications

Developing low blood pressure, especially when accompanied with correction of hypertension (high blood pressure), can lead to concerning health implications. Although these complications occur much less regularly now due to several potent blood pressure medications available, it is still necessary to understand the risk of developing these complications when treating a person with low blood pressure. Some of these complications are related to a specific cause of low blood pressure, for instance, septic shock or orthostatic hypotension. For others with similarly very low blood pressure, the complications can differ, depending on the individual and their current physicians. These complications will eventually go away once the very low blood pressure is corrected.

Angina: This is chest pain or discomfort when the heart does not obtain sufficient blood flow. Heart failure: This develops when the heart cannot pump sufficient blood to meet the body's needs. This often occurs after a heart attack or in chronic hypertension. Irregular heartbeats (arrhythmias): When the heart does not beat in a regular rhythm. Kidney failure: The kidneys cannot cleanse the blood and take away waste and extra fluids, resulting in heart failure. Persistent (chronic) hypertension can result in kidney failure. Endocrine System: The glands cannot obtain sufficient blood flow leading to glandular failure in addition to thyroid damage. Brain Effects: Insufficient blood to the brain which can result in passing out, nonreversible brain damage, or inattentiveness. Furthermore, the brain needs to have a certain pressure to keep blood from congested veins in the brain. Millions of people take 'warfarin' to make blood thin. Warfarin, in turn, increases the risk of subdural hematomas.

Chapter 4: Diagnosis and Evaluation

In clinical practice, the most important way of diagnosing and evaluating low blood pressure is for clinicians to gain a comprehensive understanding of the patient's presence and feeling. Generally, we should have three assessments: one for blood pressure, another for blood pressure-related symptoms, and the third is to examine whether the patient has a primary disease.

Measurements of the Sitting BP. The first step in diagnosing low blood pressure is to measure the patient's resting blood pressure.

Evaluating the Autonomic Function. This examination may involve a Valsalva maneuver or a deep-breathing test to monitor heart rate changes. The patient may also take a tilt test, where they lie on a special table and are quickly moved from a lying-down position to an upright position to assess a possible drop in blood pressure after standing up.

Measurement of Fluctuation of BP. Some evaluation of blood pressure fluctuation during a day or night procedure of BP measurement is required. It is typically performed using ambulatory blood pressure monitoring (ABPM) or home BP measurements.

The guideline recommends such evaluation in the low BP research, including the diagnosis and the treatment.

Assessments for Blood Pressure-related Symptoms. It is important to ask the following four questions: (1) Is there any presence of low BP-related symptoms? (2) If they felt worse at one time than any other time, what did they do or what is a useful treatment at that time? (3) Concerning a complaint, what is a relieving factor? (4) Concerning a complaint, what is an agitating factor?

Measurements of the Four Clinical Criteria by Physicians. 1. Surveys for the Presence or Absence of Heart Disease. 2. Disease State Inquiry Concerning High Blood Pressure. 3. Blood Test Items. 4. The Metabolism-Related Clinical Criteria.

When we get the results of these items and exclude the possibility of primary diseases, we may diagnose the apparent cases to be "unexplained due to previous treatment" or the cases in which "the blood pressure went down after beginning/continuing the treatment."

Medical History and Physical Examination
Approach to the patient
The approach to the patient with low blood pressure includes four major steps: a detailed medical history, a comprehensive physical examination, laboratory studies, and appropriate adjunctive and confirmatory testing. A comprehensive approach provides both immediate information and a proactive direction for the remaining clinical care. Prompt and continuous reassessment of the causes and associated findings should be part of the inpatient care plan.
Medical history
Patients should be interviewed during periods of orthostasis, if present, to verify their orthostatic versus baseline blood pressure, as well as to uncover symptoms suggestive of orthostasis, such as light-headedness, dizziness, or syncopal and presyncopal symptoms. Cau-

sation of overt syncope by hypotension or hypertension demands detailed attention. This includes an assessment of factors or complaints witnessed before or after the event, such as associated chest pain, palpitations, bladder or bowel incontinence, tongue biting, or tonic phase limb activity. The patient's posture, such as supine, sit-up, or upright, can also be informative. A review of the autonomic-sympathetic integrity, as well as daily activities, also provides insights. Photopsias, floaters, and cobwebs can indicate dry eye, retinal detachment, or other visual concerns. Tinnitus may indicate hearing loss, while epistaxis may signal recent or longstanding hypertensive control issues and hypoadrenalism. Dry skin and hair can signify adrenal insufficiency; females may present with menstrual concerns due to decreased corticosteroid hormone production by the adrenals, mainly cortisol. Weight changes, such as due to a wreck or airborne trauma, are also highly relevant. Tattle-tailing expiration due to airflow restriction indicates chronic obstructive pulmonary disease. Pain over a band that decreases when seated can be related to amyloidosis. Difficulty swallowing would be consistent with a multinodular goiter. Signs of old intravenous lines in many cases signal endocarditis. Within the medical history, it is important to probe prior medications, such as those taken for pain, mental health, or avoiding pregnancy, which can lend further background about pathophysiological causes. Antipsychotics, levodopa and sol, vasodilatory agents, have been shown to be linked to hypotension in differing patients. In addition, a dental review is encouraged, as systemic or local dental infection can trigger low blood pressures or result in permanent damage.

Diagnostic Tests

Many kinds of diagnostic tests are available to diagnose hypotension and determine its underlying cause. For clinicians to gain a clear understanding of the diagnostic process, general assessments and investigations will be described according to cause.

Most people with hypotension can be diagnosed clinically by their healthcare provider. In people who present with signs or symptoms of BP reduction such as dizziness or syncope, particular attention should be given to a recently started new drug that may have hypotensive properties. A history of dehydration, loss of blood, or gastrointestinal bleeding should be sought in volume-depleted individuals. Those with orthostatic intolerance should undergo a head-up tilt test that confirms their susceptibility to hypotension. A physical examination is necessary to identify the signs of volume depletion, such as dry mucus membranes, tachycardia, and flat neck veins. Laboratory tests of the kidneys should be performed for older people with hypotension.

There are numerous tests available for diagnostic purposes. However, among the tools employed by clinicians, standardized guidelines for testing have not been developed, so that physicians cannot utilize them to confirm the diagnosis or to assess the extent of a hypotensive condition, especially one of orthostatic hypotension. Central hypoventilation is indicated in those with hypotension who also demonstrate severely decreased $P(vCO2)$ and/or a subsequent lack of augmented $V(E)$ in response to hypotension.

Chapter 5: Treatment Options

Treatment options: Lifestyle changes that can help to treat low blood pressure include drinking more fluids, wearing compression stockings, reducing the intake of carbohydrates, increasing the salt intake, and standing up slowly. One can also be asked to eat smaller and low carbohydrate, multiple low meals per day throughout the day to prevent severe symptoms. A doctor can recommend taking certain medications such as fludrocortisone, midodrine, or pyridostigmine. These medications typically help to increase blood pressure by acting differently on different systems within the body.

Treatment Options For most people with low blood pressure, symptoms can be relieved by making lifestyle changes, which in turn can also decrease the risk of developing other chronic medical conditions. Keep in mind that treatment for low blood pressure varies depending on the cause, and whether some medications or treatments will work for one individual and whether they may stop working over time. The human body is a complicated system. Multiple things in the body need to work together in order to maintain sufficient blood flow. For this reason, even large clinical trials have trouble studying low blood pressure and its treatment in large populations over a period of time. Current recommendations call for a multifaceted approach towards the treatment of low blood pressure; treatment for one aspect should not be confused with treatment for all aspects. You may be asked to add in lifestyle changes, such as increasing fluid and salt intake, eating smaller meals, and wearing compression stockings.

Lifestyle Changes

Lifestyle changes can be especially important in older adults who are more inclined to hypotension, as well as hypertensives with concomitant low blood pressure values. Before treating these individual groups with either prescription or nonprescription medicine, the initiation of various practical lifestyle habits is indicated to influence blood pressure favorably. The American Heart Association, American College of Cardiology, and several other professional groups have actively encouraged lifestyle changes to manage high (hypertensive) blood pressure. Furthermore, nonpharmacologic interventions are also recommended by professional guidelines for non-orthostatic or uncomplicated hypotension: promote sodium and fluid intake and moderate alcohol consumption.

There is a clinical association between hypotension, autonomic neuropathy, and cardiovascular disease in the 80 million Americans with a relatively common form of low blood pressure called orthostatic hypotension (about 50% have a neurogenic form), and persons with orthostatic hypotension are also more likely to have generalized hypotension. An individual with hypotension as his or her primary complaint should begin with the simple, conservative measures usually recommended if high (hypertensive) blood pressure has not been diagnosed. Measures that may favorably influence orthostatic hypotension include sitting on the side of the bed for 1-2 minutes prior to arising, keeping the head of the bed elevated 10 to 20 degrees, avoiding carbohydrate-laden meals that result in splanchnic vasodilation, increasing salt intake, and the use of compression stockings.

Medications

Several types of medications can be used to treat low blood pressure. Pharmacologic treatment will depend on the underlying cause, but a patient's symptoms will likely be addressed. Simply using medications to raise blood pressure with no regard to the underlying cause is not generally recommended. First-line therapy would involve simple lifestyle modifications like increasing salt and water intake, using support hose, and standing up more slowly. Most of the drugs used to treat low blood pressure are also used to treat high blood pressure. Unlike high blood pressure, low blood pressure that is only a problem when you go from lying down to standing up or after eating is not typically treated. You should talk to your doctor especially if you have symptoms. Medication treatment for low blood pressure with standing up usually involves drugs that increase blood pressure by various mechanisms.

1. Fludrocortisone (Florinef or generic) is the most commonly used first-line therapy for orthostatic hypotension. It is also the first-line therapy for low blood pressure without an orthostatic component when low blood pressure leads to symptoms. This medication helps retain salt and water which can be helpful in raising blood pressure. It takes a few days or up to a couple of weeks to work. 2. Midodrine (ProAmatine or generic). This is an alpha agonist that can stimulate the blood vessels to produce vasoconstriction (squeezing the blood vessels to keep blood in them and raising blood pressure). Data on its safety and effectiveness is strong and it is used quite extensively. The biggest drawback of midodrine is that it can only be taken during the day and is associated with a number of side effects

such as a burning or tingling feeling in the scalp. The FDA requires all patients to do tilting studies to show that they have some form of blood pressure issues that would be amenable to midodrine before it is prescribed.

Chapter 6: Prognosis and Management

Individuals with chronic asymptomatic hypotension do not have any predisposing factors for the development of presyncope or syncope. However, when syncope or presyncope is present, the prognosis is determined by the primary disease. High mortality is found in individuals with postural hypotension, especially in the elderly. Significantly severe hypoperfusion symptoms are in the best prognosis.

Treatment of hypotension is still a major problem today, and there is a lack of management guidelines. The prognosis and management of hypotension vary from case to case depending on the daily activities and social norms of the patient. Acute management is very similar to chronic management and includes reversal of the state of hypoperfusion, fluid and electrolyte replacement, complete blood count, specific drug infusion, management of the underlying cause, and additional other approaches in terms of patient fluid status. The principle of treatment of hypotension includes oral and intravenous hydration (except for cardiogenic shock), removing nitrate medications, initiating and optimizing vasoactive and ionotropic support medications, and if there is a need to use adrenal corticosteroids, inotropic agents, and specific adrenergic and dopamine receptor agonists, especially in refractory shock. Ongoing management should be used.

Long-Term Outlook

This section is going to focus on the prognosis of low blood pressure and how the condition might change over time. Click on the headings below to scroll down for more information.

How Long Does It Take for Low Blood Pressure to Go Away?

Low blood pressure does not have a cure. If you have it, you can use self-care techniques and, if required, medicine for treatment. These treatments will help manage symptoms and improve your quality of life. Your blood pressure may fluctuate over time. Various factors influence blood pressure, and they may change depending on the circumstances you are in. If you have an underlying medical condition that causes your low blood pressure, it may improve if you can treat the main problem. Discuss treatment options with your healthcare provider. He or she can provide the support and guidance needed to help manage this condition effectively.

Dizziness, weakness, fainting, and fatigue may also be symptoms of low blood pressure. If you have low blood pressure, you can minimize these symptoms by applying self-care treatments and, if necessary, using medications. If you work with a healthcare professional to manage the problem, these therapies can also improve your overall quality of life. Low blood pressure can induce another underlying condition or worsen an existing condition in some situations. If left uncontrolled, low blood pressure may have these long-term effects.

Tips for Managing Low Blood Pressure

Low blood pressure can cause complications and impacts a substantial part of the population. Whenever possible, I encourage my patients to self-implement lifestyle strategies to help regulate blood pressure naturally rather than relying solely on blood pressure-lowering medication. Here are some of my tips for managing low blood pressure.

Drink water: Dehydration reduces blood volume, leading to a drop in blood pressure. Follow a diet called DASH (Dietary Approaches to Stop Hypertension): This diet, rich in fruits, vegetables, healthy fats, and whole grains, has been clinically shown to help regulate blood pressure in just two weeks. Eat small, frequent meals: Eating smaller meals with healthy snacks, such as fruit or nuts, every few hours rather than two or three large meals daily can help regulate your blood sugar level and decrease potential light-headedness due to low blood pressure. Increase your sodium: Eat enough salt or increase sodium-rich foods in your diet. Drink caffeine: Although caffeine can lead to a temporary spike in blood pressure, it can have a favorable effect on your blood pressure over the long term.

Elevate yourself: Elevate the head of your bed. Alternatively, lie down and lift your legs just above your heart. Consult with a physical therapist for help with exercises that target leg strengthening and blood pressure regulation. You might also want to cross your legs, tighten your thighs, and flex your feet when standing. Consider riding: Discuss with your doctor the possibility of taking a medication that could help increase your blood pressure. Always use caution, and never take these drugs without first consulting with a doctor. Monitor your blood pressure at home: Regularly checking your blood pressure at home can provide a sense of control and help you know if your blood pressure medication is working. Ask your doctor if home blood pressure monitoring is appropriate for you and, if so, how best to conduct it.

CHAPTER 8

Chapter 7: Conclusion and Future Directions

In summary, maintaining an optimal blood pressure is fundamental for securing life. A low blood pressure doesn't attract attention of many people because some people think that it is not life-threatening danger and it doesn't induce health's disorder consequences. Moreover, it receives less attention than hypertension from physicians. In fact, obviously low blood pressure is found less often than hypertension. Nevertheless, despite its low prevalence, the consequences of low blood pressure for health are serious and potentially fatal. The increasing health's disorder of low blood pressure that affects the life's quality of the people induced us to perform a survey to discuss this subject. We revised the literature about low blood pressure around the body, mainly the consequences for heart and brain strokes. In the future, we must run many studies concerning the parameters that are linked with low blood pressure.

We must find new treatment strategies for cardiovascular diseases and elucidate the mechanisms that may explain the tight linkage between low blood pressure and clinical affection. Potential future fundamental research into low blood pressure could include the aging process and changes in lifestyle. Large prospective studies are needed to elucidate the association between blood pressure and not only cardiovascular events and their complications. Clinical and pre-clinical studies must be performed to elaborate the mechanisms that could explain these relationships. In conclusion, several advances regarding the physiology of hemodynamics of low blood pressure, and their clinical consequences are needed to refine our knowledge about this concept.

www.ingramcontent.com/pod-product-compliance
Lightning Source LLC
Chambersburg PA
CBHW020347180726
47991CB00021B/3057